PCOS MANAGEMENT COOKBOOK FOR WOMEN

A Complete Medical Guide with Over 20-Deiting Recipes for PCOS

TABLE OF CONTENT

Every young lady dreams of becoming a mother so that she can nurture a family and share in her children's growth and happiness. No one ever considers the possibility that they might be among the infertile or that this might not happen to them. The lives of millions of women in the United States experience this every day.

The most common endocrine disorder affecting women of reproductive age (from puberty to menopause) is polycystic ovarian syndrome (PCOS). Polycystic ovarian syndrome (PCOS) is a hormonal disorder that impacts a woman's fertility and overall endocrine system health.

High levels of testosterone production, insulin resistance, obesity, hirsutism, and cardiovascular disease may all be linked to this condition.

Have been exposed to many stories and teaching methods concerning PCOS.

And in this book, I will be talking at length about polycystic ovary syndrome and providing practical guidance for coping with the condition.

Hearing the stories of people who have suffered from polycystic ovary syndrome (PCOS) is always terrible, but the most recent person I heard from particularly stuck with me since she has had PCOS since she was 11 years old.

Hearing her story brought me a lot of pain, and knowing that many other women had gone through something similar only made it worse.

Despite having had symptoms of polycystic ovary syndrome (PCOS) since she was 11 years old, Rachel just recently received a diagnosis of PCOS when I first met her. I was surprised, and I admire her determination. Even though this is the way things are, you should not hide the fact that you are healthy; instead, reassure everyone around you.

One in ten women of childbearing age suffer from polycystic ovary syndrome (PCOS). It can strike at any time after puberty, although it is often not diagnosed until a person is in their twenties or thirties and experiencing infertility. You should know this vital truth regarding PCOS. Problems with ovulation and pregnancy can be caused by PCOS.

Listening to Rachel's narrative, which outlined the difficulties she had on a daily basis due to PCOS symptoms, and then being able to give her with long-term solutions to help her better regulate those symptoms, was a tremendous blessing for me.

Is it feasible that the fact that she got her first period when she was only 11 years old is to blame for the excessive monthly bleeding and painful periods she is always endured?

At this age, the onset of menstruation is pretty common. She told me that she did not remember being in a lot of pain during this time, but that her mother sometimes had to pick her up from school because she was unprepared for her period and bled through her pants.

Rachel's periods were extremely irregular and far out, but she showed no other symptoms, so her mother assumed they will normalize once she reached high school. Still, she could not dispute that she was the only one in her social group who was having a hard time. Does this seem about right? Rachel began to have serious second thoughts.

The symptoms that Rachel was having did not improve and, if anything, were much worse. She gained weight and had painful periods as symptoms.

Her menstrual cycles were also very unpleasant. Her self-esteem plummeted as a result. Since she was considerably heavier than her peers, it was concluded that she had a weight problem.

Rachel's menstrual cycle came only once every three to four months, but it caused her excruciating pain and severe anemia each time. They thought it was strange due of her active lifestyle, which they both shared.

But this did not explain why I was in such excruciating pain or why I was bleeding so heavily. She was in such much discomfort on the first day of her period that she had to stay home from school and stay inside all day.

Rachel told me that she had to accept and work around the symptoms in order to have a normal life.

Her teachers and coaches were very kind and would let her go home without punishment on the first day of her cycle when she was unable to perform properly.

This further proves that she struggled with it back in high school. This is when I first met her, and it was during this moment that I was able to convince her that everything will turn out fine.

Even while attending university, she must keep her health condition a secret, and she must do everything in her power to ensure that no one notices.

After strictly adhering to my instructions, she felt less pain and experienced less severe bleeding. You, as a person with PCOS, must remember that there is no single method in which the disorder presents itself throughout a person's lifetime.

Therefore, in this book, I will do my best to offer you with the best methods to manage and control your PCOS symptoms through eating so that you can live the best quality of life possible.

Even though you may be familiar with PCOS in general, I always enjoy providing a brief medical lecture on the topic before diving into the meat of the matter. Refresh your memory and learn again.

A hormonal imbalance in women can lead to polycystic ovary syndrome (PCOS), also called polycystic ovarian syndrome. The ovaries are affected by the hormonal imbalance.

Every month, a mature egg is produced by the ovaries and discharged as part of a normal menstrual cycle.

Ovulation dysfunction and abnormal egg development are both symptoms of polycystic ovary syndrome.

Menstrual cycles disrupted by polycystic ovary syndrome (PCOS).

Infertility (the inability to conceive a child) has been linked to irregular menstrual cycles. PCOS is a major contributor to female infertility. Furthermore, ovarian cysts (fluid-filled sacs) may form as a result.

You should be aware that PCOS affects between 5% and 10% of women of childbearing age (15–44). In their twenties and thirties, when they have trouble conceiving and visit a doctor, most women learn they have polycystic ovary syndrome.

However, PCOS can occur at any time after adolescence. Women of all racial and ethnic backgrounds are susceptible to developing polycystic ovary syndrome. In addition, being overweight or having a mother, sister, or aunt who has PCOS may increase your risk of developing PCOS.

Type of PCOS

In order to effectively treat PCOS and reverse symptoms naturally, you need to know the type of PCOS you're dealing with. The four types of PCOS include:

Insulin Resistant PCOS

About 70 percent of all cases of PCOS fall into this category. Hyperinsulinemia, or insulin resistance, occurs when the body's cells become resistant to the effects of insulin.

This occurs when insulin's effects on our cells get dulled, prompting the pancreas to secrete ever-increasing amounts of the hormone in the hopes that our cells will finally wake up.

Weight problems, especially those centered around the abdomen, sugar cravings, and other symptoms including weariness and mental fogginess are common in this form of PCOS.

Problems like excess hair, male pattern hair loss, and acne are all linked to elevated androgen levels, which are caused by elevated insulin levels.

HbA1c and glucose tests are commonly used by clinicians, although they only provide partial information regarding a patient's blood sugar levels.

Testing your fasting insulin is the only way to confirm or disprove the presence of insulin resistance. Fasting insulin levels below 10 mIU/L (60 pmol/L) are considered normal.

To help treat insulin resistant PCOS, the key is down to improving your insulin sensitivity.

You can work on this through:

- Regular exercise and movement throughout the day helps your body to burn sugar, build muscle and improve your sensitivity to insulin.

- Avoiding high sugar foods and having a lower carbohydrate diet that is also rich in protein and fat to balance blood sugar levels.

- Prioritizing sleep and reducing stress can also help to manage blood sugar and insulin levels.

- Supplementation of key nutrients such as magnesium, chromium, NAC, inositol and berberine can also be extremely helpful.

I strongly advise working with a naturopath to find out what is best for you at what dosage, as this will vary from person to person and is key to getting results.

Post-Pill PCOS

After discontinuing oral contraceptives, some women develop PCOS. These women did not suffer from preexisting conditions like acne, menstrual irregularities, or excessive hair growth before using the pill. Because of the nature of the synthetic progestins used, oral contraceptives like Ginet, Yasmin, and Yaz are frequently associated with this kind of PCOS.

The classic PCOS signs, such as an increase in androgens after stopping the pill, are present in this form of the disorder even while insulin resistance is absent.

This usually occurs between three and six months after my customers have stopped using the medication.

It is important to remember that this type can take time to heal on its own, but can be handled more rapidly with the correct nutrition, lifestyle modifications, supplementation, or herbal medicine support.

To help treat post-pill PCOS:

- Be patient. This type can take some time to reverse, but remember it is a temporary situation.
- Speak to a practitioner about supplementation. Nutrients such as magnesium, vitamin E, vitamin B6, zinc as well as specific herbs like chaste tree and peony can be helpful to support ovulation and lower excess androgens.

- Prioritize sleep and stress management. Like insulin resistance PCOS, it is important to get a good quality sleep and reduce stress levels to support overall hormonal balance.

Adrenal PCOS

About 10% of women with PCOS have the kind caused by a misbalanced response to stress. In most cases, just DHEA-S (another adrenal androgen) will be raised, without also seeing increases in testosterone or androstenedione. Unfortunately, this form of androgen is rarely evaluated without going through an endocrinologist or another type of professional.

To help treat adrenal PCOS:

- Manage stress. Reducing stress levels through activities like yoga, meditation, mindfulness and journalling will help to support your nervous system and your hormones.

- Get enough sleep each night. Make sure you're getting at least 8 hours of sleep each night to support your stress levels and recovery.
- Avoid high intensity exercise. Limit excessive and high intensity training as this can further put a stress on your adrenals.
- Avoid caffeine from coffee, tea and fizzy drinks.

Speak to a practitioner about herbs and supplements. Specific herbs like withania, rhodiola and liquorice can help the body adapt and recover from stress. Nutrients like magnesium, vitamin B5 and vitamin C are also important to support the adrenal glands and nervous system.

You'll need to speak to a professional about correct dosages and which supplements to take, especially when it comes to herbs as they may not be right for you.

Inflammatory PCOS

Overproduction of testosterone and associated clinical symptoms are hallmarks of inflammatory polycystic ovary syndrome (PCOS). Symptoms of inflammation in this kind of PCOS include headaches, joint discomfort, unexplained exhaustion, skin disorders like dermatitis, and gastrointestinal symptoms like irritable bowel syndrome.

Blood tests often reveal elevated inflammatory markers, such as a C reactive protein (CRP) level above 5. However, inflammation can occasionally cause readings for tests like fasting glucose and insulin to fluctuate slightly outside of the usual range.

To help treat inflammatory PCOS:

- Address gut health. Repairing leaky gut tissue, balancing gut bacteria, improving digestive enzymes and eliminating pathogenic bacteria are all important steps to reduce overall inflammation.

- Remove food triggers. Addressing potential food sensitivities and removal of inflammatory foods is a vital step to help address inflammation. It can sometimes be quite difficult to figure out what foods might be driving your inflammation, so it's best to work with a nutritionist on this who can help you.

- Natural anti-inflammatories such as turmeric , omega 3 fatty acids as well as antioxidants like NAC can help to support this type of PCOS.

Always speak to a practitioner first to see if these are right for you, and in what dosages to take them for them to be effective.

COULD IT BE SOMETHING ELSE?

Hypothalamic amenorrhea is a disorder that is sometimes misdiagnosed as polycystic ovary syndrome. Hypothalamic amenorrhea (HA) is when you stop having periods and it can be brought on by things like not eating enough or exercising too much.

Ultrasound findings consistent with polycystic ovary syndrome (PCOS) have been linked to HA as well as similar acne and hair growth symptoms. The treatment for the two illnesses is different enough that an inaccurate diagnosis becomes a problem.

The fundamental difference between PCOS and hypothalamic amenorrhea is the ratio of follicle-stimulating hormone (LH) to ovarian follicle-stimulating hormone (FSH).

A higher than normal ratio of luteinizing hormone (LH) to follicle stimulating hormone (FSH) is associated with polycystic ovary syndrome (PCOS). On the other side, LH levels can be significantly lower than FSH levels in women with hypothalamic amenorrhea.

Some of the symptoms of PCOS include:

- ### **Irregular menstrual cycle**

if you have PCOS you may miss periods or have fewer periods (fewer than eight in a year). Or, your periods may come every 21 days or more often. Even Some women with PCOS stop having menstrual periods.

- You can have too much hair on your face, chin, or parts of the body where men usually have hair. This is called hirsutism. Hirsutism affects up to 70% of women with PCOS.

- Acne on the face, chest, and upper back

- Thinning hair or hair loss on the scalp; male-pattern baldness

- Weight gain or difficulty losing weight

- Darkening of skin, particularly along neck creases, in the groin, and underneath breasts
- Skin tags, which are small excess flaps of skin in the armpits or neck area

The exact cause of PCOS is not known. Most experts think that several factors, including genetics, play a role but some of the major causes are;

- **<u>High levels of androgens</u>**

Androgens are sometimes called "male hormones," although all women make small amounts of androgens. Androgens control the development of male traits, such as male-pattern baldness.

Women with PCOS have more androgens than normal. Higher than normal androgen levels in women can prevent the ovaries from releasing an egg (ovulation) during each menstrual cycle, and can cause extra hair growth and acne, two signs of PCOS.

- ## **<u>High levels of insulin</u>**

Insulin is a hormone that controls how the food you eat is changed into energy. Insulin resistance is when the body's cells do not respond normally to insulin. As a result, your insulin blood levels become higher than normal.

Many women with PCOS have insulin resistance, especially those who have overweight or obesity, have unhealthy eating habits, do not get enough physical activity, and have a family history of diabetes (usually type 2 diabetes).

Over time, insulin resistance can lead to type 2 diabetes.

With the aspect of talking about your mensuration, you might be wondering can you still get pregnant if I have PCOS. Yes of course! Having PCOS does not mean you can't get pregnant.

PCOS is one of the most common, but treatable, causes of infertility in women. In women with PCOS, the hormonal imbalance interferes with the growth and release of eggs from the ovaries (ovulation). If you don't ovulate, you can't get pregnant.

And also know that PCOS is linked to other health problems including:

Diabetes: More than half of women with PCOS will have diabetes or prediabetes (glucose intolerance) before the age of 40.

<u>High blood pressure:</u> Women with PCOS are at greater risk of having high blood pressure compared with women of the same age without PCOS. High blood pressure is a leading cause of heart disease and stroke. Learn more about heart disease and stroke.

<u>Unhealthy cholesterol:</u> Women with PCOS often have higher levels of LDL (bad) cholesterol and low levels of HDL (good) cholesterol. High cholesterol raises your risk of heart disease and stroke.

<u>Sleep apnea:</u> This is when momentary and repeated stops in breathing interrupt sleep. Many women with PCOS have overweight or obesity, which can cause sleep apnea. Sleep apnea raises your risk of heart disease and diabetes.

<u>**Depression and anxiety:**</u> Depression and anxiety are common among women with PCOS.

Also know that at menopause your **PCOS** symptoms may or may not go away because **PCOS** affects many systems in the body and from different women with **PCOS** that have work with i find that their menstrual cycles become more regular as they get closer to menopause. However, their **PCOS** hormonal imbalance does not change with age, so they may continue to have symptoms of **PCOS**.

<u>**Endometrial cancer:**</u>

Problems with ovulation, obesity, insulin resistance, and diabetes (all common in women with PCOS) increase the risk of developing cancer of the endometrium (lining of the uterus or womb).

And also, the risks of PCOS-related health problems, such as diabetes, stroke, and heart attack, increase with age. These risks may be higher in women with PCOS than those without.

PCOS Diagnosing Procedure

There is no single test to diagnose PCOS. To help diagnose PCOS and rule out other causes of your symptoms, your doctor may talk to you about your medical history and do a physical exam and different tests:

Physical exam

Your doctor will measure your blood pressure, body mass index (BMI), and waist size.

They will also look at your skin for extra hair on your face, chest or back, acne, or skin discoloration.

Your doctor may look for any hair loss or signs of other health conditions (such as an enlarged thyroid gland).

Pelvic exam

Your doctor may do a pelvic exam for signs of extra male hormones (for example, an enlarged clitoris) and check to see if your ovaries are enlarged or swollen.

Pelvic ultrasound (sonogram)

This test uses sound waves to examine your ovaries for cysts and check the endometrium (lining of the uterus or womb).

Blood tests

Blood tests check your androgen hormone levels, sometimes called "male hormones." Your doctor will also check for other hormones related to other common health problems that can be mistaken for PCOS, such as thyroid disease. Your doctor may also test your cholesterol levels and test you for diabetes.

Once other conditions are ruled out, you may be diagnosed with PCOS if you have at least two symptoms I mentioned above.

PCOS Treatment

Don't let anyone scam you if they tell you they have a cure. No! There is no cure for PCOS, but you can manage the symptoms of PCOS. I have help a lot and am happy at last am writing this book. In chapters to come I will explain the key reason why this book is best for you.

The fundamental steps you can take at home to help relieve your symptoms include;

Losing weight

Healthy eating habits and regular physical activity can help relieve PCOS-related symptoms.

Losing weight may help to lower your blood glucose levels, improve the way your body uses insulin, and help your hormones reach normal levels. Even a 10% loss in body weight (for example, a 150-pound woman losing 15 pounds) can help make your menstrual cycle more regular and improve your chances of getting pregnant.

Removing hair

You can try facial hair removal creams, laser hair removal, or electrolysis to remove excess hair. You can find hair removal creams and products at drugstores.

Procedures like laser hair removal or electrolysis must be done by a doctor and may not be covered by health insurance.

Slowing hair growth

A prescription skin treatment (eflornithine HCl cream) can help slow down the growth rate of new hair in unwanted places.

In vitro fertilization (IVF)

IVF may be an option if medicine does not work. In IVF, your egg is fertilized with your partner's sperm in a laboratory and then placed in your uterus to implant and develop.

Compared to medicine alone, IVF has higher pregnancy rates and better control over your risk of having twins and triplets (by allowing your doctor to transfer a single fertilized egg into your uterus).

<u>**Surgery**</u>

Surgery is also an option, usually only if the other options do not work. The outer shell (called the cortex) of ovaries is thickened in women with PCOS and thought to play a role in preventing spontaneous ovulation.

Ovarian drilling is a surgery in which the doctor makes a few holes in the surface of your ovary using lasers or a fine needle heated with electricity. Surgery usually restores ovulation, but only for 6 to 8 months.

In terms of using medicines, the types of medicines that treat PCOS and its symptoms include;

Hormonal birth control: including the pill, patch, shot, vaginal ring, and hormone intrauterine device (IUD). If you a woman who don't want to get pregnant, hormonal birth control can make your menstrual cycle more regular and lower your risk of endometrial cancer

Anti-androgen medicines: These medicines block the effect of androgens and can help reduce scalp hair loss, facial and body hair growth, and acne.

They are not approved by the Food and Drug Administration (FDA) to treat PCOS symptoms. These medicines can also cause problems during pregnancy.

Metformin

Metformin is often used to treat type 2 diabetes and may help some women with PCOS symptoms. It is not approved by the FDA to treat PCOS symptoms.

Metformin improves insulin's ability to lower your blood sugar and can lower both insulin and androgen levels. After a few months of use, metformin may help restart ovulation, but it usually has little effect on acne and extra hair on the face or body. Recent research shows that metformin may have other positive effects, including lowering body mass and improving cholesterol levels.

How PCOS affect pregnancy

PCOS can cause problems during pregnancy for you and for your baby.

Women with PCOS have higher rates of:

- Miscarriage
- Gestational diabetes
- Preeclampsia
- Cesarean section (C-section)

You can lower your risk of problems during pregnancy by:

- Reaching a healthy weight before you get pregnant. Use this interactive tool to see your healthy weight before pregnancy and what to gain during pregnancy.

- Reaching healthy blood sugar levels before you get pregnant. You can do this through a combination of healthy eating habits, regular physical activity, weight loss, and medicines such as metformin.

- Taking folic acid. Talk to your doctor about how much folic acid you need.

PCOS can be difficult to navigate alone. Remember that it is a complex hormonal disorder that can take time to resolve. If you're tired of being on hormonal contraception, are looking to start a family, or would just like to manage your PCOS symptoms naturally.

CHAPTER TWO

PCOS DIETING AND LIFESTYLES

Coping with polycystic ovarian syndrome (PCOS) or its symptoms can be quite frustrating at times. Irregular periods or no menstruation at all, acne, excessive hair growth, insulin resistance, and difficulty losing weight are just some of the things on your list of woes. If uncontrolled, PCOS can lead to serious complications such as high blood pressure, heart disease, diabetes, and endometrial cancer.

What you eat or don't eat can play a significant role in influencing the severity of your PCOS symptoms. Many women with PCOS have been able to reduce their risk of medical complications and better manage their symptoms by making positive changes in their diet.

What you eat plays a massive role in deciding the health and condition of your body. It is because the type of food you eat triggers different hormones. That is true in the case of people who suffer from PCOS.

Those who suffer from PCOS have higher levels of insulin than average. Insulin is a hormone released by the pancreas that helps break down glucose and turn it into energy used by the body. If your body lacks insulin, glucose doesn't break down, causing your blood sugar level to rise.

However, the situation is the opposite in people affected by PCOS. They have high portions of insulin in their blood. When the amount of insulin in the blood increases, the ovaries produce higher levels of androgens.

Increased insulin in the blood can also cause the body mass index to rise and make it difficult to lose weight.

Diet Do's and Don'ts for PCOS

Do's

Do have more of high-fiber foods

They slow down the digestive process and reduce sudden increases in blood sugar levels which helps in combatting insulin resistance. Broccoli, cauliflower, red and green peppers, almonds, sweet potatoes, and pumpkin are great examples of high-fiber foods.

Do have more of lean proteins

Although they do not have much fiber, lean-protein foods such as chicken, fish, and egg whites keep you feeling full longer and help stabilize your blood sugar.

Do have more anti-inflammatory foods

Inflammation is part of the underlying mechanism of PCOS and foods with anti-inflammatory properties which include tomatoes, spinach, strawberries, walnuts, almonds, turmeric, and fatty fish such as sardines and salmon help to reduce the symptoms of PCOS.

Don'ts

Don't have refined carbohydrates

Foods such as white breads, pastries, muffins, and white potatoes exacerbate insulin resistance and cause inflammation which will worsen your PCOS symptoms.

Don't have sugary snacks or drinks

Excess sugar is one of the main causes of insulin resistance and should be avoided at all costs. When checking food labels, look for the other names of sugar such as sucrose, dextrose, and high fructose corn syrup.

Don't have inflammatory foods

These foods exacerbate PCOS symptoms. Foods such as French fries, margarine, red meat, and other processed meats belong to this group and should be avoided as much as possible.

Foods for PCOS Diet
What to eat

Foods high in fibre and protein or help reduce inflammation could be good additions to a PCOS diet. They can help ease symptoms of PCOS to a large extent.

Some foods that are high in fibre content are:

Cruciferous vegetables: These may include broccoli, Brussels sprout, cabbage, cauliflower, radish and so on.

Leafy greens: These may include arugula, Chinese chard, collards, Dandelion greens, kale, mustard greens, rapini, Swiss chard

Reens and red peppers: These are composed of 92% water. In addition, they have a variety of vitamins and minerals that are very useful for the body.

Beans and lentils: As per research, beans and lentils are a rich source of fibre and protein. They have many other benefits like better heart health and reduced blood sugar levels.

You can include protein sources in your diet as well. They are very filling and an excellent dietary option. Examples of protein sources include;

- Tofu
- Chicken
- Fish
- Eggs

- Dairy products

In addition, you could add various foods to your diet that are proven to reduce inflammation. Some of the options are:

- Tomatoes
- Kale
- Spinach
- Walnuts
- Olive oil
- Fatty fish

What you avoid

You should avoid foods that have refined carbohydrates. There are various reasons for avoiding such foods. Research suggests that refined carbohydrates increase the risk of inflammation, which can cause obesity.

Further research in this area indicates that it can drive you to eat more, a significant cause of obesity worldwide.

Examples of foods having refined carbohydrates include:

- White bread
- Muffins
- Pastries
- Sugary desserts
- Fries
- Margarine

Lifestyle Changes

There are various lifestyle changes that you can adopt if you have PCOS. Though most lifestyle changes will not treat PCOS directly, they will help manage the symptoms that accompany PCOS.

Regular Physical Activity

Physical activity improves metabolism, blood flow, heart health, and lung strength and elevates overall mood. It can also help you lose weight (as being overweight is a common problem in PCOS).

You can include physical activities like walking, jogging, running, swimming, cycling, dancing, weight training or any other activity that requires you to move. You can consistently do it just a few days per week to see the results.

Adequate Sleep

Various studies have shown that lack of sleep is strongly related to hormonal imbalance. Taking adequate sleep of 7-9 hours per day is associated with multiple benefits and can help ease various symptoms of PCOS.

A good sleep is vital to losing weight. Being overweight is a common problem in PCOS, so this benefit is critical. For example, adequate sleep can reduce the chances of type 2 diabetes, reduced cases of depression and create a good overall mood.

Avoid Smoking and Alcohol Consumption

If you have PCOS, you are already at a greater risk of high blood sugar levels and diabetes. Avoiding smoking will help you prevent lower blood sugar levels. That raises blood sugar levels and increases the risk of diabetes. Similarly, alcohol consumption is associated with an increase in blood sugar levels.

Check Out for Symptoms of Depression

Studies suggest that people suffering from PCOS are more likely to face symptoms of depression. So PCOS symptoms should seek out support from health groups to ease the symptoms. If necessary, they should consult a therapist as well.

Low-Carb Breakfast Recipes

With the sea of information of nutrition information, it can quickly feel overwhelming to plan nutritious, healthy breakfasts to support your PCOS.

The thing is, it doesn't have to be complicated. There are lots of foods you can incorporate into your PCOS-friendly breakfast, and many do not take more than a few minutes.

Breakfast Waffle Sandwich

Serves: 4

Prep Time: 5 Mins   Cook Time:: 30 Mins

Ingredients

To assemble

- 4 breakfast sausage patties (see notes)

- 6 large eggs

- 2 tablespoons milk

- 1/4 teaspoon kosher salt

- 2 tablespoons butter + more for butter

- 1/8 teaspoon ground black pepper

- 4 slices cheese, American, cheddar, pepper Jack

For the waffles

- 1 cup all-purpose flour

- 1 teaspoon baking powder

- 1/2 teaspoon kosher salt

- 1 cup milk

- 1/4 cup unsalted butter, melted

- 1 large egg

Directions

- Preheat your oven to 400 degrees. Place the sausage patties on a small baking sheet and bake for

15-20 minutes until browned and cooked through.

- Meanwhile, preheat your waffle iron. A mini waffle iron works best but a large square waffle iron would work as well.

- To prepare the waffle batter, whisk together the flour, baking powder, and salt in a medium bowl. Add the milk, melted butter, and egg and stir until just combined. There should still be some small lumps.

- Ladle 1/4 cup of waffle batter into mini waffle iron or 1 cup into a large square waffle iron and cook for 2-3 minutes until the waffles are set and begin to brown just slightly. Repeat with the remaining batter.

- Heat a medium non-stick skillet over medium-low heat. In a bowl or a liquid measuring cup, whisk together six eggs with two tablespoons of milk, 1/4 teaspoon kosher salt, and 1/8 teaspoon ground black pepper. Melt two tablespoons of butter in the skillet and swirl it to coat. Add the eggs and allow to cook undisturbed for about 30 seconds, then use a spatula to lift and fold the eggs. Cook for another 15 seconds then repeat, lifting and folding until the eggs are softly set. This should take about 2 minutes total. Remove from heat and set aside.

- Heat a large skillet, preferably cast-iron, over medium-low heat.
- Layer three of the waffles with a sausage patty, then scrambled eggs and a slice of cheese before topping it with another waffle.

- Butter the outer side of each sandwich and transfer the sandwiches to the hot skillet and cook on each side for about 2-minutes, until golden and crispy. Remove from heat and serve warm with syrup if desired. **If you used a large square waffle iron, you will need to cut the waffles into four portions for a total of eight.

Protein Waffle

Serves: 1

Prep Time: 2 Mins

Cook Time:: 5 Mins

Ingredients

- ½ Cup Protein powder
- 1 Egg
- 3 Tablespoons Plain fat free Greek Yogurt or sour cream
- 1 teaspoon Baking powder
- pinch of salt

- butter and sugar free syrup for serving

Directions

- Heat your waffle iron on medium and spray with cooking spray.
- Mix the protein powder, egg, Greek Yogurt, baking powder, and salt in a medium sized bowl until fully combined.
- Pour half of the batter in the waffle iron (for smaller waffle irons, pour less batter), and cook according to your waffle irons directions.
- Serve with butter and sugar free syrup.

Ingredients

- 2 ripe bananas
- 2 large eggs
- 1 teaspoon vanilla extract
- ½ teaspoon baking powder
- 1 teaspoon baking soda
- ½ teaspoon cinnamon
- ⅛ teaspoon nutmeg
- Pinch of salt
- 2 cups almond flour
- ¼ cup cashew nuts roughly chopped
- ¼ cup pumpkin seeds
- ¼ cup semi-sweet chocolate chips

Directions

- Preheat the oven to 350°F. Line a muffin tin with 9 muffin liners.

- In a food processor, blend the bananas, eggs, vanilla, baking powder, baking soda, nutmeg powder, cinnamon, nutmeg, and salt at medium speed until combined.

- Add the almond flour to the banana mixture and blend until well combined, scraping down the sides with spatula as necessary.

- Using an ice cream scoop or two large spoons, drop the mixture evenly into the muffin liners.

- Sprinkle the muffins with cashews, pumpkin seeds, and chocolate chips.

- Bake for 20 minutes, or until a toothpick inserted into the center of a muffin comes out mostly clean.

Let the muffins cool on a cooling rack.

Maple Low Carb Oatmeal

Serves: 4

Prep Time: 5 Mins

Cook Time:: 20 Mins

Ingredients

- 60 g (½ cups) walnuts
- 60 g (½ cups) pecans
- 40 g (¼ cups) sunflower seeds
- 15 g (¼ cup) coconut flakes
- 1000 ml (4 cups) unsweetened almond milk
- 4 tbsp (4 tbsp) chia seeds
- ⅜ tsp (⅜ tsp) stevia powder
- ½ tsp (½ tsp) cinnamon
- 1 tsp (1 tsp) maple flavouring (optional)

- Add the walnuts, pecans and sunflower seeds to a food processor and pulse a few times to crumble them up.

- In a large pot, add all of the ingredients. Put on low and simmer for a good 20-30 minutes, stirring, until the chia seeds have absorbed most of the liquid. Don't forget to stir as the seeds can stick to your pot at the bottom!

- When the oatmeal has thickened, turn off the heat and serve hot. You can also let it cool down and store it in the fridge for your breakfast the next day.

- Serve with fresh fruits and any other desired toppings

Prep Time: 15 Mins   Cook Time:: 50 Mins

Ingredients

- 1 10oz. box frozen chopped spinach
- 8 oz. mushrooms
- 1 clove garlic, minced
- 1/8 tsp Salt
- 1 Tbsp cooking oil, divided
- 2 oz. feta cheese
- 4 large eggs
- 1/4 cup grated Parmesan
- 1/4 tsp pepper
- 1 cup milk
- 1/2 cup shredded mozzarella

Directions

- Preheat the oven to 350°F. Thaw and squeeze as much moisture out the spinach as possible.

- Rinse any dirt or debris from the mushrooms, then slice thinly. Mince the garlic.

- Add the mushrooms, garlic, salt, and a ½ Tbsp cooking oil to a skillet. Sauté the mushrooms over medium heat until they have released all of their moisture and it has evaporated from the skillet. No water should remain in the skillet.

- Brush the other ½ Tbsp cooking oil inside a 9-inch pie plate. Layer the mushrooms, spinach, and crumbled feta into the pie plate.

- In a large bowl, whisk together the eggs, Parmesan, pepper, and milk.

- Pour the egg mixture into the pie plate over the spinach, mushrooms, and feta. Top with the shredded mozzarella.

- Bake the crustless quiche in the preheated 350°F oven for about 50 minutes, or until it is golden brown on top and the internal temperature reaches 160°F. Slice and enjoy!

Chicken & Apple Sausage Sweet Potato Hash

Serves: 5

Prep Time: 15 Mins   Cook Time:: 24 Mins

Ingredients

- 1 Tbsp. ghee or coconut oil
- 3 strips Applegate No Sugar Uncured Bacon, cut into ¼–½ inch pieces
- 1 medium sweet potato, peeled and cut into small cubes (~2 cups)
- 2 cups halved Brussels sprouts
- 1 small zucchini, sliced or diced
- 1 small red pepper, sliced
- ½ small red onion, sliced or diced

- 1–2 Tbsp. fresh thyme leaves (or 1 tsp. dried), optional
- 4 Applegate Chicken & Apple Sausages, sliced (¼-inch slices)
- Salt and pepper to taste

Directions

- In a large cast iron skillet or pan, heat ½ Tbsp. ghee or coconut oil on medium-high heat. Once hot, add cubed sweet potato, Brussels sprouts and bacon. Dash with salt and pepper and sauté for about 12 minutes. Stir occasionally, adding additional ghee or oil as needed.
- Next to the pan, add the zucchini, red pepper, onions, sausage and optional thyme. Sauté for 10-12 minutes or until sweet potatoes and Brussels sprouts are cooked through. Again, adding additional ghee or oil as needed.

- Serve just as it is or you can serve it over top of greens and with a fried egg on top.

Smothies Recipes

Avocado Berry Fertility Smoothie

Serves: 1

Total Time: 5 Mins

Ingredients

- ½ cup zucchini chopped and frozen
- ½ banana frozen
- ½ cup berries frozen
- ¼ avocado
- 1 tbsp almond butter (or alternate nut butter)
- 1 cup spinach
- 1 cup almond milk (or alternate milk)
- ½ cup whole milk yogurt, plain

- Add all ingredients to blender and process until creamy.
- If more sweetness is desired, feel free to add sweetener of choice to taste.

Low-carb Banana Spinach Smoothie

Serves: 1

Total Time: 5 Mins

Ingredients

- 1½ cups fresh spinach
- 1 cup unsweetened almond milk
- ¼ cup frozen banana
- ¼ cup frozen avocado
- ¼ cup plain Greek yogurt
- 2 tsp chia seeds
- ½ tsp vanilla extract
- 1 scoop vanilla protein powder

Direction

- Add frozen banana, frozen avocado, spinach, chia seeds, vanilla extract, almond milk, and Greek yogurt to the blender. Blend for 30 seconds to a minute, until no spinach shreds remain.

- Add protein powder, and pulse 4-5 times until combined. Serve!

Papaya Creamsicle Smoothie

Serves: 1

Total Time: 5 Mins

Ingredients

- ½ ripe medium papaya
- 4 oz. fortified 100% orange juice
- 4 oz. unsweetened almond milk
- 1 scoop vanilla protein powder
- 3-4 ice cubes (optional)

- After washing the outside of the papaya and slicing it in half, scoop out the seeds with a spoon and discard. Then, scoop out the flesh from one half and add it to a blender.

- Add orange juice, almond milk, and protein powder. Add some ice cubes if desired for a colder, refreshing temperature. Blend well- about 30 seconds.

- Garnish with a slice of orange and enjoy!

Banana Almond Butter

Serves: 1

Total Time: 5 Mins

Ingredients

- 1 c spinach

- ½ c of 5% Fage plain yogurt

- 1 small banana

- 1 tsp of cinnamon
- 2 tbs of almond butte
- 1 c of unsweetened vanilla almond milk

Directions

- Add everything to the blender and blend on high until smooth. For a thicker smoothie add ice.

Chocolate Peanut Butter Banana Serves: 1

Total Time: 5 Mins

Ingredients

- 1 c of unsweetened vanilla almond milk
- 1 c of spinach
- 1 small banana
- 2 tbs of peanut butter
- 1 tbs of chia seeds
- 1 tsp of cinnamon

- 1 scoop of protein powder

Directions

- Add everything to the blender and blend on high until smooth. For a thicker smoothie add ice.

Salad

Tomato., Cucumber and Red Onion Salad

Ingredients

- 2 large cucumbers, peeled and coarsely chopped
- 3 large tomatoes, coarsely chopped
- 2/3 cup red onion, coarsely chopped
- 1/3 cup balsamic vinegar
- 1/2 tbsp white sugar
- 3 tablespoons extra virgin olive oil
- Salt and pepper, to taste

- Fresh basil or mint leaves, for garnish (optional)

- In a large bowl with a lid, combine all ingredients. Cover, and shake to mix.
- Season with salt and pepper.

Beet and Carrot Salad with Ginger

- 1/2 cup raw beets, peeled and grated
- 1/2 cup organic carrots, grated
- 2 tbsp apple juice
- 1 tbsp extra-virgin olive oil
- 1/2 tsp fresh ginger, minced
- 1/8 tsp sea salt

- Combine grated beets and carrots in a small bowl.
- Mix apple juice, olive oil, ginger, and salt in a separate bowl and drizzle over salad mixture. Toss gently. Enjoy!

Arugula, Avocao and Tomato Salad

Ingredients

- 3 cups young arugula leaves, rinsed
- 2 cups cherry tomatoes, halved
- 1/4 cup sun-dried tomatoes, chopped
- 2 tablespoons extra virgin olive oil
- 1 tablespoon balsamic vinegar
- 2 small avocados, peeled, pitted and sliced

- In a large plastic bowl with a lid, combine arugula, cherry tomatoes, sun-dried tomatoes, olive oil, and vinegar. Toss well.

- Divide onto plates, and top each serving with slices of avocado.

Chicken and Apple Salad

Ingredients

- 3 cups cooked chicken, diced
- 1 cup grapes, halved
- 1/2 cup celery, diced
- 3 tbsp red onion, finely chopped
- 1/2 cup organic apples, diced
- 6 tbsp extra light mayonnaise
- 2 tsp lemon juice
- Salt and pepper, to taste
- Lettuce leaves

- Combine first five ingredients in a large bowl.

- In a small bowl, combine mayonnaise, lemon juice, and salt and pepper. Stir into chicken mix.

- Arrange lettuce leaves on serving plates and top with chicken salad.

Dinner

Cripsy Chicken Sald with Honey Mustard Dressing

Serves: 4

Prep Time: 20 Mins   Cook Time:: 15 Mins

Ingredients

Honey Mustard Dressing

- ¼ cup honey

- ¼ cup mayonnaise homemade or store-bought (I like Primal Kitchen)

- ¼ cup Dijon mustard (yellow mustard will work too)

- 1 tablespoon lemon juice or white distilled vinegar

Fried Chicken

- 1 lb chicken tenderloins (Note 1 chicken breasts)
- 2 large eggs
- ½ cup all-purpose flour gluten-free if needed
- ¼ cup Panko breadcrumbs gluten-free if needed
- 1 teaspoon garlic powder
- ½ teaspoon paprika (I like smoked paprika)
- 1 teaspoon salt
- ¼ teaspoon black pepper
- ⅓ cup coconut or avocado oil plus more if needed

Crispy Chicken Salad

- 8 cups romaine lettuce chopped

- 3-4 hard boiled eggs quartered (Note 2)
- 1-2 avocado sliced or chopped
- ½ red onion thinly sliced
- 1 cup cherry tomatoes halved

Directions

- Start by making the salad dressing. Add all of the ingredients to a small dish and whisk until smooth. Place in the fridge until ready to serve.
- To make the crispy chicken salad, pat the chicken tenders dry with a paper towel and season both sides with kosher salt and pepper
- Create a dredging station with three shallow bowls large enough to fit each chicken tender. Add ¼ cup of flour to the first bowl then whisk the eggs in the second bowl. To the third bowl, whisk together the remaining

¼ cup of flour, Panko bread crumbs and seasoning.

- Line a large plate or baking sheet with parchment paper to place each piece of dredged chicken. Using one hand, place a chicken tender in the bowl of flour and turn to coat it on both sides. Transfer it to the bowl of beaten eggs to coat, then cover it in the panko mixture last. Turn it to coat well to ensure all sides are covered in breading. Transfer the chicken to the prepared plate or pan and repeat with the remaining tenders. Your fingers will be coated in the mixture, but it's best to wait until you're done with all of the tenders before washing them.

- To fry the chicken, pour the oil into the bottom of a large, deep skillet, like a cast iron skillet, over medium-high heat. Use an instant-read thermometer to determine when the oil is hot enough to add the chicken. The oil should reach 325°F before adding the chicken.

- When the oil is up to temperature, place half of the chicken tenders in the oil. Check the temperature of the oil again, doing your best not to touch the thermometer to the bottom of the pan to get an accurate reading. The oil temperature will drop when you add the cold chicken, so adjust the heat as needed to keep the temperature as close as you can to 325. Fry the chicken for approximately 4 minutes on each side, until the breading is golden brown and the internal temperature of the thickest part of the chicken reaches 160°F (just under the target temperature of 165°F), to allow for carryover cooking.

- When the chicken is done, transfer it to a paper towel line plate and repeat with the second half of the chicken. Allow the chicken to cool and rest while you assemble the salad.

- Add the lettuce to a large bowl and top with hard-boiled eggs, sliced avocado, red onion, cherry tomatoes, and cheese if desired. Slice the chicken into large chunks or strips and top the salad. Serve with prepared dressing.

Creamy Cajun Chicken Pasta

Serves: 8

Prep Time: 10 Mins   Cook Time:: 20 Mins

Ingredients

<u>*For the cajun seasoning*</u>

- 2 teaspoons smoked paprika
- 1 teaspoon oregano
- 1 teaspoon dried thyme
- ½ teaspoon garlic powder
- ½ teaspoon onion powder
- ¼ teaspoon cayenne pepper
- ¼ teaspoon black pepper
- ¼ teaspoon salt
- or 1 tablespoon cajun seasoning

<u>*For the chicken pasta*</u>

- 1 lb boneless skinless chicken breast
- 14 ounces pre-cooked smoked sausage cut into slices (look for no sugar added) I like Aidell brand
- 2 tablespoons olive oil
- 1 medium yellow onion diced
- 12 ounces gluten free penne pasta brown rice or chickpea pasta

- 14.5 ounce can fire roasted tomatoes
- 2 cups chicken broth or bone broth
- ½ cup coconut cream
- Chopped parsley or green onion for topping

- If making your own seasoning, combine the ingredients for the cajun seasoning in a medium bowl. If you're using premade seasoning, add it to a medium bowl. Set aside.
- Cut the chicken into ½ inch cubes and add to the medium bowl with the cajun seasoning. Toss to coat the chicken evenly in the seasoning using a wooden spoon. Set aside.
- Add the olive oil to the bottom of a deep skillet over medium-high heat and allow to heat for a few minutes until the oil is rippling. Add the

seasoned chicken to the skillet and cook for 1-2 minutes on each side to brown the sides. The chicken doesn't need to be cooked all the way through yet.

- Add the diced yellow onion and smoked sausage to the pan with the chicken and continue to cook, stirring frequently, until the onion is soft and translucent, about 2-3 minutes.

- Add the penne pasta, fire roasted tomatoes with the juice and the broth to the chicken, sausage and onions. Stir until everything is combined then close the lid of the pan and allow it to come to a boil over medium-high heat.

- Once boiling, turn the heat down to medium-low and let the pasta simmer for about 10 minutes, stirring every few minutes. If you're using a chickpea pasta, pay attention to the pan as it tends to foam. When it's done the mixture should be thick and saucy and the pasta should be tender.

- Add the coconut cream to the pan and mix until melted and combined.

Sheetpan Garlic Herb Streak and Potatoes

Ingredients

For the potatoes

- 1 ½ lbs mixed baby potatoes halved

- 2 tablespoons olive oil

- 4 garlic cloves minced

- 1 teaspoon thyme chopped

- 1 teaspoon rosemary chopped

- ½ teaspoon dried oregano

- Salt and pepper to taste

For the steak

- 1 ½ pound flank steak

- 2 teaspoons garlic powder

- 1 teaspoon Italian seasoning

- 1 teaspoon paprika

- ½ teaspoon crushed red pepper flakes

- 1 teaspoon salt

- ½ teaspoon black pepper

- Parsley for topping

For the caramelized onion (optional)

- 1 tablespoon coconut oil or olive oil

- 1 large yellow onion sliced

- Preheat oven to 400°F. Line a large baking sheet with foil or spray with non-stick cooking spray.

- If you're making caramelized onion, add coconut or olive oil to a medium saucepan over medium heat. Add the sliced onion, and cook, stirring frequently, for 15-20 minutes or until the onions soften and turn a dark amber color.

- Add the halved baby potatoes to the pan and drizzle with 2 tablespoons olive oil. Top with minced garlic, thyme, rosemary, dried oregano, salt and pepper. Toss well to coat the potatoes. Roast in the preheated oven for 20 minutes, stirring halfway through.

- While the potatoes are roasting, prepare the steak. In a small bowl, combine the garlic powder, Italian seasoning, paprika, red pepper flakes, salt and pepper in a small bowl. Season steak by rubbing the spice mix on both sides.

- When the potatoes are ready, remove from the oven and turn the oven to broil mode. Stir the potatoes and push them to one side of the pan. Place the seasoned steak on the opposite side and place back in the oven. Broil the steak for 5-7 minutes on one side then remove from the oven, flip the steak, stir the potatoes and place back in the oven. Broil the other side of the steak for another 5-7 minutes or until medium rare (135°F).

- Remove from the oven and sprinkle with parsley and top with caramelized onion if using.

Prep Time: 10 Mins   Cook Time:: 25 Mins

Ingredients

- 5-6 medium zucchini (2 1/4-2 1/2 pounds total), trimmed
- ¾ teaspoon salt, divided
- 1 ripe avocado
- 1 cup packed fresh basil leaves
- ¼ cup unsalted shelled pistachios
- 2 tablespoons lemon juice
- ¼ teaspoon ground pepper
- ¼ cup extra-virgin olive oil plus 2 tablespoons, divided
- 3 cloves garlic, minced
- 1 pound raw shrimp (21-25 count), peeled and deveined, tails left on if desired
- 1-2 teaspoons Old Bay seasoning

Directions

- Using a spiral vegetable slicer or a vegetable peeler, cut zucchini lengthwise into long, thin strands or strips. Stop when you reach the seeds in the middle (seeds make the noodles fall apart). Place the zucchini "noodles" in a colander and toss with 1/2 teaspoon salt. Let drain for 15 to 30 minutes, then gently squeeze to remove any excess water.

- Meanwhile, combine avocado, basil, pistachios, lemon juice, pepper and the remaining 1/4 teaspoon salt in a food processor. Pulse until finely chopped. Add 1/4 cup oil and process until smooth.

- Heat 1 tablespoon oil in a large skillet over medium-high heat. Add garlic and cook, stirring, for 30 seconds. Add shrimp and sprinkle with Old Bay; cook, stirring occasionally, until the shrimp is almost cooked through, 3 to 4 minutes. Transfer to a large bowl.

- Add the remaining 1 tablespoon oil to the pan. Add the drained zucchini noodles and gently toss until hot, about 3 minutes. Transfer to the bowl, add the pesto and gently toss to combine.

Roasted Red Bell Pepper Soup

Serves: 6

Prep Time: 15 Mins   Cook Time:: 24 Mins

Ingredients

- 3 red bell peppers
- 1 onion, chopped
- 1 tablespoon minced garlic
- 1 tablespoon olive oil

- 2 (15 ounce) cans cannellini beans, drained and rinsed
- 2 (14.5 ounce) cans chicken broth
- salt and pepper to taste

Directions

- Preheat oven to broil.
- Place the bell peppers on a baking sheet and broil on the top rack of the oven, using tongs to turn them as each side blackens. Place the blackened peppers in a paper bag, close tightly and allow them to cool for 20 to 30 minutes. Then peel the skin off the peppers and discard the stem and all the seeds. Chop the peppers and set aside.
- In a large pot over medium heat, saute the onion and garlic in the oil for 5 minutes, or until onion is translucent. Now add the chopped,

roasted red bell peppers and saute for 2 to 3 more minutes.

- Next, add the chicken broth and the beans, stirring well. Using a blender, puree the soup in small batches and return to the pot over low heat for 5 minutes.

Salmon & Cauliflower Rice Bowl

Serves: 2

Prep Time: 15 Mins   Cook Time:: 20 Mins

Ingredients

- 2 salmon fillets, sustainably sourced or organic
- 10 to 12 Brussels sprouts, chopped in half
- 1 bunch kale, washed and shredded

- ½ head cauliflower, pulsed into cauliflower rice (you can use a whole cauliflower head if you wish)
- 3 tablespoons olive or coconut oil
- 1 teaspoon curry powder
- Himalayan salt

For marinade

- ¼ cup tamari sauce
- 1 teaspoon Dijon mustard
- 1 teaspoon sesame oil
- 1 teaspoon honey or maple syrup (optional)
- 1 tablespoon sesame seeds

Directions

- Preheat oven to 350°F.
- Line a baking tray and add chopped Brussels sprouts. Coat with 1 tablespoon oil and season with salt. Add to oven and roast for 20 minutes.

- Meanwhile, make marinade by combining all ingredients in a bowl and whisking until combined.

- Remove Brussels sprouts after 20 minutes and add salmon fillets to the baking tray. Spoon marinade over salmon fillets and return to oven for a further 13 to 15 minutes, or until salmon is cooked to your liking.

- While salmon is cooking, heat a pan over medium-high heat and add 1 tablespoon oil. Add kale and sauté until wilted (2 to 3 minutes). Remove from pan and set aside.

- Heat remaining oil in pan and add cauliflower rice. Season with 1 teaspoon curry powder and salt and sauté until cooked (2 to 3 minutes).

- Remove salmon and Brussels sprouts from oven and divide into

two bowls. Add sautéed kale and
cauliflower rice to bowls.

Never lose the hope! Never agree to the fact that PCOS can hold you down. This is your breakthrough therefore hold this guide thigh and high!.